Children Healing:

40 Effective Recipes for Kids' Health

TABLE OF CONTENTS

Introduction

I would like to thank and congratulate you for downloading *"Healing Children Naturally: Natural Remedies for Kids!"* I can assure you that you will feel much better in knowing that these remedies for common ailments are made with natural ingredients that will not cause any harmful side effects to your child. There is no artificial additives or ingredients in these remedies. Too many synthetic drugs or medications in the world come with many bad side effects. With many of them often causing more discomfort to the person than the ailment they are supposed to be treating.

Like most parents, you want the best for your child, and that includes the kinds of treatments that you provide for them when they are ill. The immune systems of children in general are lower than adults, so they are often more prone to sore throats, colds, stomach aches, and various other illnesses. Choosing to use homeopathic medicines is an excellent choice, as they are a much safer alternative compared to many over the counter drugs and their undesirable side effects. Because they are a safer choice, many parents are opting to choose natural remedies for their children's illnesses.

Chapter 1. Natural Remedies for Children

When you are seeking remedies to treat your child's ailments such as sore throats, stomach aches, and colds, your doctor will even tell you that the old-fashioned home remedies work the best for common ailments. These natural remedies have been tried and tested over many years, and have proven their effectiveness. They have a history of working fast, and rarely come with any side effects and are very affordable. Most people can afford these natural remedies, many of the ingredients for them you may already have.

There have been scientific studies proving the safety and effectiveness of some of the more common natural remedies for example ginger and chamomile. If your child is suffering from a serious condition, you need to take them to see a doctor to get a proper diagnose of their ailment. However, if it is minor aches and ailments you are dealing with then you can easily take care of them using these homemade remedies.

Chamomile tea for colic
Using chamomile tea to help the intestinal muscles of infants to relax works well, it is known to help children also to calm down according to many pediatricians. You can steam the tea for 5-minutes before you allow it to cool. Transfer about 2-ounces of it to a baby bottle and then give it to your baby. Do not give your baby more than 4-ounces in a single day, to give you baby enough space for breast milk and formula.

Cayenne Pepper to help stop nosebleeds
Cayenne pepper will help to clot blood, studies have revealed that this remedy has been used by many cultures around the world, it is nothing new. While you apply, this make sure that your child's head is upright before you pinch his nostrils together for a few minutes. You can then sprinkle the cayenne pepper on a piece of moistened cotton swab which you can dab inside your child's nose. A pinch of cayenne pepper is enough, dab it

on the area that is bleeding. You might be worrying thinking that this sounds like it will sting, but it doesn't and it will stop the bleeding.

Honey & Lemon Juice

Use this combination to treat your child's sore throat. The lemon will work to dry up the congestion while the honey will offer a nice soothing coating. Studies have shown that giving a child a spoonful of honey works better than cough medicine. You can combine one tablespoon of lemon juice and one tablespoon of honey and put it into the microwave for 2 minutes to warm up. After it has warmed up give it to your child, one teaspoon at a time. Do not give this to babies under 1 year old, honey is not safe for them.

Baking soda for treating bug bites

It has been reported that parents that have used this remedy have stated that it works better and faster than store bought products. There is alkaline in baking soda that helps to counteract the acidic swelling. You can mix about one teaspoon of baking soda with some water until you create a thick paste. Smear this paste on the bug bites and leave it on to dry. This will help to stop the itching.

Duct tape for warts

Warts can be very difficult to get rid of, but using the gray fabric of duct tape works well as they cannot resist it and it hinders their growth. If your child suffers from warts place a small piece of duct tape over the affected area but do not put it on too tight so that it causes discomfort to your child. When the tape begins to get tattered change it. If you do this for about a month you will get rid of the wart.

Contact lens solution to help reduce congestion

This remedy can be used on children over 6 months. Use a saline solution free of preservatives inside a syringe to help reduce your child's congestion. Ensure that their head is raised before you gently squeeze the solution into their nostrils. It is best to do this over a bath or sink. Recent studies have shown that a mixture of sea water and nasal wash was important in helping kids to recover faster from colds and reduced their chances of getting sick again.

Using a sock to treat tummy or neck pain

The next time that your child experiences tummy or neck pain, you can create a heat wrap using a sock and filling it with uncooked rice before tying it closed using a string. Place the sock in a microwave for about 1 minute and let it become warm. Then place it on the area that it affected, when it cools down place it back into the microwave. Do this until the pain disappears.

A bubble wand to cure anxiety

Children also suffer from stress, you can find ways to help alleviate it. Normally, a child can relax by breathing slowly and deeply according to pediatricians. To make this process a bit more effective you can give your child a soapy wand to breathe into and blow length and unhurried streams of bubbles from it.

Treat car sickness with fresh ginger tea

There are kids who get nauseous when they travel in vehicles such as cars. There is a natural remedy for this. It is best used on children over 2 years of age. Some honey can make it taste a lot more appealing to a child. After you boil the ginger tea, allow it to cool before you give it to your child to drink. Give this to your child about 30 minutes before they get into the vehicle. The ginger in the tea will stop the contractions and your child will not get car sick. The contractions are what normally convince your child's brain that they are feeling sick and nauseous.

Use a credit card to help with a bee sting

If your child is stung by a wasp or bee it is advisable to remove the stinger to avoid the wound becoming infected with extra venom. Many people try to squeeze the stinger, but this is not advisable because it can cause the venom to spread. What is advised is that you use the flat edge of your credit card to scrap it off. Do this over the sting and only stop when the stinger has come out.

Use cucumber to stop mild swelling

You may have observed that spas will use cucumber slices to place over client's eyes to help to reduce the puffiness around eyes. This is done because cucumber can soothe hot swollen skin. After slicing the cucumber place one slice on the area of minor swelling. Have a couple of slices in the fridge so that when the one on the injury get warm you can replace it with a new cold slice of cucumber.

Remedies for children's tummy problems

Most children will have tummy problems at one point or another. You can help solve this problem by using a slippery elm tincture. Mix a couple of drops of it in some water and let your child drink it. It will take about 10 minutes for the tummy ache to disappear, it will help with gas too. You can find non-alcohol tincture in most health food stores, that you can carry with you when you travel. Using a glycerin based option is recommended. Use it according the instructions on the bottle. You can also try a warm bath or a wheat bag to help relieve a tummy ache.

Help ease child's indigestion with a stick of gum

This remedy is suggested for use by children 4 years or older. If your child is complaining of a full stomach, after consuming a large meal then give them a stick of gum. The act of chewing the stick of gum will produce extra saliva which is an important part of the process of neutralizing the excess acid in the stomach which could be giving your child problems according to gastroenterologists.

Remedy for pink eye

To stop pink eye, you can use raw milk or colostrum to treat it. A drop or two will be enough. If you find that your child gets pink eye frequently, this is a sign that they have a vitamin A deficiency and taking cod liver oil a daily can also help.

Remedy for Diarrhea

To help remedy diarrhea, broth is the best at stopping it. The best way to administer this to your child is a few tablespoons at any given time, this can be done more frequently. Broth contains gelatin that will help to bind the liquid found in the colon. Once the liquid becomes bulky it will stop coming out as diarrhea and will help to control the loss of fluids. If it is a case of severe diarrhea you might want to try enema this will also counteract dehydration as well.

Remedy for vomiting

If your child is vomiting you should not give them any water or food for the next two hours. Doing this is only going to make your child's situation worse. It can be hard to do this, as often after vomiting a child will feel thirsty. It is best to wait two hours before you give them any liquids. If your child becomes extremely thirsty you might want to try giving them an ice-cube to suck on, though it still is not wise. You can also try giving them diluted juice using a bulb syringe.

Remedy for boils

Boils can often make parents panic, but they are another way that the body uses to eliminate toxins. It is not a wise choice to give your child antibiotics to get rid of boils. You instead can try mixing chickweed, tomato slices, cooked onions, gently warmed cabbage leaves, crushed garlic and plantain leaves before wrapping them up and applying them as a compress on the affected area. You can use plastic wrap to cover it up, and tape the edges with surgical tape. It is important that you keep the poultice wet, it needs to be changed several times daily. When you do this the boil's head will appear and they you can use a sterilized needle to prick it and drain it and leave it to heal.

Remedy for chicken pox

The best thing you can do for your child when they have chicken pox is to let it run its course. Don't stop it, as it will help to strengthen your child's immune system. You can relieve the itching with soda baths. Use a one pound box of soda for a bath.

Remedies for whooping cough

One of the worst childhood ailments is characterized by a coughing fit that lasts about seven weeks. Children cannot go out during this time, because this ailment is contagious. You should take your child to the doctor so that they can be diagnosed properly. There are sites that deal with whooping cough online. You can record your child's cough and send it to them, they can make a diagnosis telling you whether it is whooping cough or not that your child is suffering from.

If your child is strong and healthy you can avoid antibiotics. If you do this your child could go a very long time without suffering from a cold because their immune system will be stronger. The best thing regarding whooping cough is that if your child gets it they can never get asthma. To date there are not many natural remedies for whooping cough. Some people say that Elderberry soup or Drosera help to ease the cough. These do little to help with whooping cough, including antibiotics, they basically help to avoid spread the disease. The illness must run is course, once your child begins to cough there is nothing you can do about it to stop it. You can try to alleviate the coughing fits using a HEPA filter which is very expensive. This can be placed in your child's bedroom and it will help to diminish the frequency of their coughing fits. Also have cod liver oil if your child has whooping cough, the vitamin A in it will help his/her lungs to function well.

Remedies for headaches

You can help to soothe your child's headache by simply placing a towel that is filled with ice-cubes on their forehead. Do not place the ice directly onto their skin, since it will burn. Often diet has a considerable influence on your child getting headaches and how frequent they are occurring. If a child is eating a well-balanced diet they will rarely get headaches. The reason being is they often occur when there is low blood sugar. Providing your child with three solid meals a day that include sufficient amounts of animal protein and should also be high in fat. Too much sugar in their diet can also lead to headaches. Limit your child's consumption of sugars.

Your child may get a headache after playing a physical game such as soccer, this is due to becoming dehydrated because of the exercise involved. You can rehydrate your child with coconut milk, and diverse types of fermented drinks which work better than water in this case. If your child is very active in a lot of sporting activities I would suggest having lots of canned coconut water available for their consumption during these sporting activities.

Give your child water if you do not have the above beverages, do not exceed 2 bottles that are four ounces every 30 minutes. Too much water will just go to their kidneys. They should only take green tea as a last resort for curing headaches. The green tea should be very mild and taken in lesser amounts. The tea has caffeine so when administering it to children you want to give them only tiny amounts.

Treatments for ear infections

According to research a connection has been discovered between diet and childhood infections. According to research it has been found that children who are well fed or have a good traditional diet don't get ear infections. If you are breastfeeding your child and they get an ear infection you should carefully consider your diet. Pasteurized milk is one of the things that should limit your diet because they tend to have the effect of ear infections. You can try placing a warm wheat bag on their ear. This will offer your child a great deal of relief from the ear pain. Wheat bags are normally made from fabric that has unground wheat kernels inside it and it is something that you can create yourself if you do not want to purchase one. Place it in microwave with ½ a cup of water until it becomes hot to the touch which will be about a minute or two. Place it onto your child's ear and it will offer them relief. Another option you might want to try is to add some warm olive oil by dropping it into your child's ear. You might find this difficult as children will often not want you to do this, try explaining the benefits of it to your child.

You can also try using ear candles for healing your child's ear infection. Some people are under the impression that ear candles help to clean the ear, but this is not the case. Instead, they dry out any moisture that may be present within the ears. Therefore, you can use them to blow some warm smoke inside your child's ear and stop the ear infection.

This inflammation of the outer ear, is often painful, so it is important to know how you can alleviate your child's suffering. The inflammation of the outer ear often will attract bacteria and liquid. It therefore could become infected and if this is the case it is advisable that you consult a pediatrician who will most likely prescribe an antibiotic in the form of drops. However, if it is a mild case, you can try to evaporate the water trapped in your child's ear that is causing the inflammation. You could try using a dryer, but make sure that you are not standing too close to your child. Aim the dryer at their ear and allow it to dry the water. Set the dryer to warm to avoid harming your child.

Remedies for fevers

Parents often are sent into a panic when their child develops a fever. There are things that you can do to handle the situation and the first rule of thumb is to never try to lower the fever which is the first thing that normally comes to mind. Avoid using Tylenol and ibuprofen drugs that many parents run to when a fever develops. Change your attitude towards the fever and instead of viewing it as something that is harming your child, be grateful for its existence because the existence of it means that it is performing important tasks within your child's body.

Traditionally, parents did not bring down a fever but instead they waited for it to die down because they believed that it would help to prolong the illness as well as contributing to weakening their child's ability to fight diseases, therefor making it easier for another one to attack them.

Many people believed that by bringing down the fever it would cause the sickness to worsen the next time. Studies have shown that there is a connection between repeatedly reducing childhood fever and childhood cancer. It has also been proven that a secondary infection will occur if you eliminate fever. So, by bringing down your child's fever you will be essentially starting the cycle of using antibiotics because your child's immune system will be suppressed.

It is important that you recognize that fever plays a key role in ensuring your child's overall health and wellbeing. It does this by slowing down the pathogens which are the virus or bacteria that want to cause your child pain and these multiply after every few minutes. When your child's body reacts by producing a fever, the severity and spread of the illness is slowed down. Therefore, bringing the fever down enables the virus or bacteria to spread further and attack your child's body.

When you see your child's, temperature rising there is no need to panic between 102-103 as this is the standard range for a fever. The best thing you can do it to hold and comfort your child during a fever, even if it takes hours. We often will want to monitor our children's temperature but you do not have to. You will know by placing your lips on their forehead.

There are times when a fever can take 3 days though it will not be constant and its peak time will usually be between 4-6 in the afternoon. Your child might have a fever in the afternoon, and sleep well through the night, but this does not mean the fever is over. So, it is best not to send them to school until you make sure that the fever does not return. If it does not return then you can send your child back to school. You can feel good in knowing at this point they are well on their way to full recovery.

Food can help to reduce the fever naturally, this is fine because you haven't forced it. If your child can eat, give them some food. Do not force them to eat and do not overfeed your child. If you have found that your child's fever has gone past the normal range, this is when you can attempt to bring it down. You might want to try using a cool water enema. It is not a popular form of treatment for most, especially children, but it will bring down the fever.

If the fever is too high, place a large beach towel inside the tub and lay your child on his/ her side but do not remove their clothes. Instead just slide down their pajamas a little. Place some warm filtered water inside of a bag, about ½ to 1 quart of water. After you have inserted the enema nozzle, your child will begin to feel the urge to go to the bathroom. Place your child on the toilet and allow them to use the bathroom. The fever will reduce by 1 or 2 degrees. High fevers range from 104-105 degrees, they cannot be classified as dangerous, but they are responsible for rapidly increasing the rate of metabolism and lead to the increased risk of dehydration.

During this stage, there will be a drop in the blood sugar level and this can lead to convulsions. To avoid this always keep your child hydrated during a fever. Giving them diluted fresh fruit juice can help your child stay hydrated while maintaining a normal range blood level. If your child is not able to take anything, you can try administering it using a bulb syringe. Place a few drops of cod liver oil on your child's tongue because the fever will normally deplete their vitamin A.

On the other hand, if the fever is too low, you can help to rise it by placing your child in a tub of the hottest water they can handle. Allow them to soak in the hot tub for about 12 minutes.

Get your child out of the tub and dry them as quickly as you can. Wrap them up tight and get them into bed and cover them up. The fever will rise by morning, their temperature will have gone back to normal.

Chapter 2. Natural Remedies for Your Child's Sore Throat

When our children are suffering from a sore throat, we often will seek antibiotics. The problem with this is when antibiotics get overused, this can lead to resistant bacteria in your child and therefore doctor's do not rush to prescribe them. This is the reason that there has been an increase in bacteria that is resistant to modern antibiotics over the years. This adds to the risk of potentially deadly infections.

Most sore throats are caused by viral infections not bacterial infections; therefore, antibiotics will not help in treating these sore throats. There is only a small number of sore throats that can be contributed to bacteria infections, and these are related to diphtheria, whooping cough and strep throat. There are some natural solutions that can help to treat sore throats.

Peppermint

A wonderful way to ease a sore throat and gain fresh breath at the same time by using peppermint. Peppermint sprays are great for relieving sore throats and this is according with the American Cancer Maryland Medical Center. Their studies reveal that the menthol found in peppermint is what is responsible for calming sore throats and coughs in addition to thinning mucus. In 2011, there was a study that discovered spray solution having a combination of five herbs inclusive of peppermint had more chances of improving sore throats compared to a placebo.

Peppermint contains anti-bacterial, anti-inflammatory and antiviral properties according to a study carried out in 2008 and these can help encourage healing.

If you use these natural remedies, you may have no need to see a doctor unless the symptoms worsen. When you do use, these remedies make sure that you have enough rest and drink plenty of liquids to help speed up the recovery process.

Echinacea and Sage

A combination of Echinacea and sage had been found to help reduce the symptoms of sore throat. There was a study performed on 159 patients in 2009. The patients had been experiencing sore throat for at least 12 years. These patients were given Echinacea/sage throat sprays and some received medical chlorhexidine/lidocaine spray for three days. These sprays were taken after every two hours in the form of two puffs which added up to about 10 daily. The results of the study revealed that Echinacea/sage spray worked as effectively as the medicinal spray used to treat sore throats.

Salt water

Using salt in warm water to gargle with has been known to help sooth sore throats in addition to breaking down secretions. You can use this remedy to also kill bacteria existing in the throat. This mixture can also help to reduce swelling and will ensure that the throat will remain clean.

Honey

A great and tasty home remedy for relieving a sore throat is taking some honey directly or mixing it in tea. A study including 139 children, who suffered from upper respiratory infections was carried out. The results of this study showed that honey worked more effectively at controlling nighttime coughs even compared to the common cold suppressants. Honey has also been shown to help in healing wounds, it thus helps a sore throat to heal faster.

Slippery elm

Slippery elm is a remedy that has been used traditionally for a long-time cure for sore throat. It was often used by Native Americans to provide relief from sore throats and coughs. When this remedy is mixed with water it creates a slick gel. This gel coats and soothes the throat.

Licorice Root

A sore throat is normally painful and can even prevent a child from sleeping soundly even if it is not very serious to the extent of needing a doctor's attention. The use of licorice root has been used for many years in making a gargle by mixing it with water, it helps to reduce coughing and soothes sore throats.

Chapter 3. Natural Home Remedies for Spring Allergies

During the Spring season both adults and children alike suffer from allergies. Using natural remedies can offer your child some relief of the symptoms that go along their allergies such as sneezing.

Natural histamine block
Some people have suggested success using apple cider vinegar with some nettles. It is not in general easy for children to swallow these. You might want to add a spoonful of honey to make it more bearable for them.

Raw honey
Using the raw honey remedy is one that the children will be more than willing to take. Using raw local honey to create a strong tolerance for the local allergy triggers will help it to be effective. It must be raw honey, ask honey sellers where you can purchase local raw honey. Do not use this remedy on children under 1 year old.

Neti Pot
Using a Neti pot can remove all the allergens from sinuses when warm salted water is used. It can create some strange feelings for kids, but it will work. You should use filtered or distilled water for this remedy.

Keep air fresh
Make sure that you keep your air fresh indoors. Ways you can do this include opening the windows to ventilate a room, using natural cleaning products and so on.

Avoid using fragrance

Perfumes always make allergies worse, these can be found in many assorted products such as body cream, shampoos, fabric softeners just to name a few. You should choose to use personal care products that are fragrance-free. You can also choose this option when it comes to laundry products. Laundry is another area that can cause your allergies to become aggravated.

During allergy season, it is best not to hang out bedding, as pollen can stick to wet fabric, this can trigger your child's allergies when they use the sheets that were hung outside during allergy season.

Chapter 4. Home Remedies for Flu

We all know how miserable we have felt when we were suffering from the symptoms of flu, it is even worse for babies suffering from it. These can develop in the form of fever, nasal congestion, cough, chills and aches among others. To help your child so they do not have to suffer this misery there are remedies that can help to ease the symptoms. Most often all you need is a modest home remedy in the case of mild or moderate flu symptoms.

Drink plenty of fluids

Flu will normally make one dehydrated and this is especially the case if it is accompanied with vomiting and diarrhea. You should then make sure that your child is taking sufficient fluids to avoid becoming dehydrated. Taking lots of water, fruits juices and electrolyte beverages is a clever idea. Try to avoid giving your child drinks that are filled with caffeine, as it is a diuretic. To avoid your child from throwing up, allow them to take fluids in sips not gulps. If your child's urine is a light color to almost colorless, then you are giving them the right amount of liquids.

Soups

The classic soup for treating colds and flu is 'chicken soup' used for generations by parents to treat their sick children. Research has shown that chicken soup can offer relief to upper respiratory tract infections one of these being flu.

Plenty of rest

If your child is feeling under the weather, and feels like staying in bed to continue to rest, then allow them to do so. Part of the way that your child's body can fight diseases is to have plenty of rest. Making sure that your child is getting at least a good eight hours of sleep a night is important in helping their immune system to work well.

Humidify

Breathing in moist air can help to ease both nasal congestion and sore throat pain. This is applicable to children four years of age and older. You may also prepare a steamy shower for your child for a few minutes, several times a day and allow them to inhale the steam. You can also use a humidifier. Make sure when you use a humidifier that you clean it often to prevent the accumulation of mold and mildew.

Make a tent

If you are looking for a fast way to unclog your child's airways us a pot of boiling water. Remove the pot from heat and drape a towel over your child's head. Have them lean over the top of the pot with the towel acting like a tent holding in the steamy air. Tell your child to keep their eyes closed as they breath in the air. Have them breathe through their nose for about 30 seconds. You can increase the effectiveness of this process by adding a few drops of peppermint or eucalyptus essential oils to the water in the pot. You can repeat this process until your child has gotten relief, but only do it for 30 seconds each time.

Swish and spit

Using salt water to gargle with will help get rid of thick mucus build-up in your child's throat. It will also help to ease stuffy ears.

Warm compress

If your child is suffering from sinus pain or headaches you can try using a warm compress. Place it on their forehead or nose to gain relief of headache or sinus pain.

You are your child's caregiver
Most of us when we are sick we do not feel like doing anything, this can also be said of our children. When your child has a sore throat or cold and so on, they will feel more comforted if you are there or another close family member. Tending to them during their illness by bringing them foods and fluids and tucking them lovingly into their beds will help them to feel much better. Find ways that you can make your child feel special and loved, these can help your child to gain the desire to recover.

Conclusion

I hope that you and your child will enjoy using this collection of home remedies that will help to have your child feeling right as rain in no time without the use of synthetic drugs. You will feel good in knowing that these natural remedies will not cause your child undue stress unlike many synthetic medications that are often accompanied with bad side effects. Instead allow your child to build-up their immune system naturally, so that their bodies can fight against ailments without the use of anti-biotics and medications. Using this collection of home remedies, you will be able to do just that!

I would like to thank you once again for downloading my book, your support of my work means a great deal to me. I would love to read a review of my book by you in Amazon. I wish you remarkable success with using these natural remedies to keep your child in good health!